The Prostate Massage Manual
What Every Man Needs To Know For Better Prostate Health and Sexual Pleasure

By Ronald M Bazar

The Prostate Massage Manual

What Every Man Needs To Know For Better Prostate Health and Sexual Pleasure

Ronald M. Bazar

Published by:
Ronald M Bazar, PO Box 73, Cortes Island, BC V0P 1K0 Canada

Email: healthyprostate@yahoo.com

July 2016

Medical Disclaimer

This book contains information about health. It is not intended to replace medical advice by your doctor. It is recommended that you ask your doctor about prostate massage and its suitability for you. You, the reader, are responsible and not the author for any medical outcomes that may occur as a result of applying the methods found herein.

Ronald M Bazar is the author of six other books on the prostate:

> *Healthy Prostate: The Extensive Guide to Prevent and Heal Prostate Problems Including Prostate Cancer, BPH Enlarged Prostate and Prostatitis* (Simply type the shortened URLs into your browser's address bar: goo.gl/pVZ6tr)

> *Prostate Cancer Prevention Diet* (goo.gl/gF4vjX)

> *The Prostate Health Diet* (goo.gl/0UR6Zt)

As well as the general health and diet book:

> *Your Perfect Diet: How to Customize Your Diet for Weight Loss and Great Health (goo.gl/Abjvup)*

> *Sleep Secrets — How to Fall Asleep Fast, Beat Fatigue and Insomnia and Get a Great Night's Sleep (sleepsecrets.co/)*

Table of Contents

Introduction

Prostate massage is a new world for most men.

Why?

Most of us have not learned enough about the prostate and its importance for great health in general and sexual health for men, in particular, let alone for ultimate sexual pleasure and sexual stamina.

And only a relative few of us have learned about ways to massage the prostate for health and stimulation.

Prostate massage and sexual instruction isn't something men generally talk about over beer. Let's face it! It's been a bit of a taboo topic. Thank goodness that is changing.

Some men may think that they shouldn't do prostate massage. Such thinking would be a mistake for two reasons.

1. Prostate massage, when done correctly, can be a very healthy thing to do for your overall prostate health.

2. When sexual stimulation is intentionally added to the massage, the resulting sexual male orgasm can be exceptionally powerful. Who wouldn't want that?

Western men are facing prostate problems in epidemic proportions. Every year, approximately 6.5 million American men visit doctors for an enlarged prostate. In 2014, another 233,000 will be diagnosed with prostate cancer in the USA. In the same year, over 29,000 men will die from prostate cancer.

Plus, prostate problems are not an old man's disease any more.

More and more men are dealing with prostate disease at ever younger ages. Western males are particularly at risk and are 30 to 50 times more likely of getting prostate cancer than an Asian, Indian or African man. Worse if you are African American, who have the highest rates in the world.

With stats like this, you can't take the chance of not knowing how to take care of your own prostate. Time to stop making prostate massage a taboo subject, guys!

And for the best in sexual orgasmic pleasures, your prostate is the switch that can take you on a new journey of discovery. Time to learn all about that male G-spot gland at any age, especially if you want to last longer and heal any erectile dysfunction problems you may have.

Did you know that prostate massage was practiced in ancient times by Tantric and Taoist temple priestesses, courtesans and geishas for they knew of its wonderful health benefits and pleasures for men?

For you to have optimal health, your prostate must be kept healthy. One of the best ways to do that is through prostate massage.

Look at our modern lifestyle. We sit for so many hours each day, which causes congestion in our prostate. We eat foods filled with harmful ingredients that we can't pronounce, and we use a myriad of toxic household and body care products most days.

I go into more depth about these topics in several of my other books on prostate health (*Healthy Prostate, Prostate Cancer Prevention Diet, Prostate Health Diet*), but prostate massage is something that you can be doing right now for your prostate's health.

Our prostate is one of our body's filters and it stores some of the above-mentioned toxins and stagnant fluids. If you're middle aged and you've never done prostate massage, that's years of accumulation! And our prostate is our most sensitive gland, needed for our health and sexual fulfillment.

There's no shame in taking care of your health. Therapeutic prostate massage is a very beneficial skill. It is becoming essential for better health and sex in this modern age of exposure to so many toxins.

Even if you don't have prostate problems, you might want to begin to think about what you can do to prevent these from happening to you. Prostate massage is just one simple way to maintain prostate health or to help your prostate regain its health if you have a problem.

And—an added bonus—prostate massage can open up a whole new world of incredible sexual orgasms if you are so inclined. As a side benefit, it can help alleviate erectile difficulties by strengthening the pubococcygeus or PC muscle and by stimulating the prostate erection nerves so you can get it up. It will also help minimize premature ejaculation problems by strengthening the prostate muscles giving you more control than ever before.

Prostate orgasms are way more powerful than regular orgasms. They last longer, more ejaculate is released, and your whole body thrives from the intensity.

If you suffer from erectile or sexual difficulties, then prostate massage will help to overcome the problem by increasing blood flow to the prostate area thereby strengthening the prostate and pelvic floor muscles naturally. You see, the prostate is both a gland producing secretions and a muscle that pumps ejaculate.

And if you use a specially designed prostate device, you actually squeeze the prostate further thus strengthening all the muscles that control erections. It is the prostate and its prostate erection nerves that stimulate erections not the penis when you add sexual arousal. This massage will help to get it up and keep it up longer, solving the problem at its source.

Although I direct this book to men, it is also for women who want to further understand the prostate and to learn ways to support men in their quests for better prostate health. It may also be useful to women to increase mutual sexual pleasure and to give your man explosive longer-lasting orgasms (no longer the exclusive domain of women!).

My advice is that before you start doing prostate massage, check with your doctor or healthcare practitioner to see if it is okay for you to do, especially if you have an acute prostate condition.

In this book, we will begin by learning all about the amazing functions of the prostate.

I will discuss the benefits of massage in greater detail so you can decide if it is something you want to do.

I will describe prostate exercises, which are a form of prostate massage through special exercises.

I will then describe how to do external prostate massage and finish with internal prostate massage.

Lastly, we will talk about sexual prostate massage and techniques so you can reap the rewards of incredible prostate orgasms.

All along you will be guided with exact details to do your prostate massage safely, easily and very comfortably. No pain. Just gain.

Chapter 1
The Prostate's 10 Amazing Functions

Once you learn about these 10 amazing functions, you'll understand that it's no wonder the prostate is so vital to men's health, sex and the propagation of the species. The following chapter is from my book, *Prostate Health: Learn the 10 Amazing Functions of Your Prostate*.

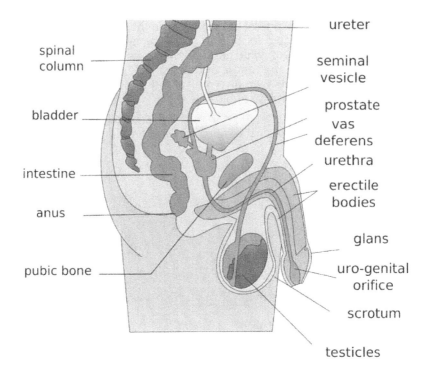

Function 1: Gland

The primary job of the prostate is to produce and secrete about 30–35% of the seminal fluids during ejaculation. Being alkaline, the prostate fluid, which is milky whitish in color, helps the sperm survive in the acidic vaginal environment. The prostate is considered to be a gland since glands secrete something.

By the way, your penis is *not* a gland as it doesn't secrete anything. It is just a superb delivery vehicle—and a fun one at that! (At least when it is working properly!)

Function 2: Mix Master

The prostate mixes its fluids with those from the seminal vesicles to transport the sperm made in the testicles. Together these fluids surge through the prostate into the urethra during ejaculation. The urethra doubles as the semen tube during ejaculation and as the urine tube from the bladder, both fluids exiting the tip of the penis. The section of the urethra that runs through the prostate gland is called the prostatic urethra and is about 3cm (1½") long.

Prostate-specific antigen (PSA) is a fluid produced in the prostate and plays a key role in enabling the sperm to swim into the uterus by keeping the semen in liquid form. PSA counteracts the clotting enzyme in the seminal vesicle fluid, which essentially glues the semen to the woman's cervix, next to the uterus entrance inside the vagina. PSA dissolves this glue with its own enzyme so that the sperm can dash into the uterus and impregnate an egg if it is there.

It is this same PSA that is tested during the PSA blood test, a very controversial test because of the many factors that can cause the results to vary widely.

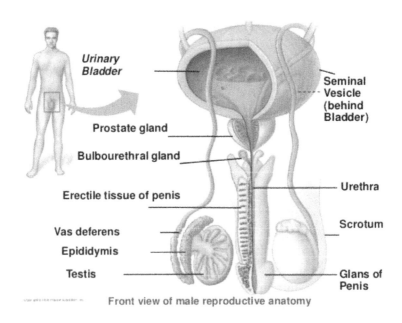

Front view of male reproductive anatomy

Function 3: Muscle

The prostate is also a muscle that pumps the semen out through the penis with enough force to enter into the vagina to help the sperm succeed in reaching the cervix and to help ensure procreation of the species.

Function 4: AH!

An added bonus for males—the pumping action of the prostate sure feels good, making sex desirable and thus helping procreation.

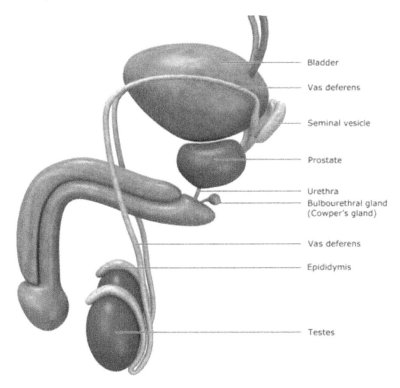

That's the prostate under the bladder...

The 2 little sacks on the right of the bladder are the seminal vesicles that produce about 60% of the seminal fluid that is pushed into and through the prostate when you ejaculate. The prostate adds another 30-35% of the total ejaculate. Those gonads or testicles (testes) produce the sperm.

Function 5: Male G-Spot

The prostate is the male G-spot. Prostate stimulation can produce an exceptionally strong sexual response and intense orgasm in men that are receptive to this sexual technique.

The ability to control ejaculation with the prostate can also lead to prolonged orgasms and "injaculations" when no semen is expelled. This is done in advanced Taoist and Tantric sexual practices to contain the sexual energy internally. If you want to learn more about this see the Resources section at the end of the book.

Strengthening the prostate gland's muscles by doing prostate exercises helps with sexual function, erection control and ejaculation mastery.

Function 6: Filter

The prostate also filters and removes toxins for protection of the sperm. Healthy sperm enhance the chance of impregnation and ensure that men seed with robust sperm.

This is perhaps the prostate's most important function and, at the same time, can be one of the main reasons for the growing epidemic of prostate disease and cancer as men deal with more and more toxins in food and the environment.

If you can't remove those same toxins from your prostate gland, they accumulate and can begin to create prostate disease. Yes, your lifestyle choices have something to do with waking up multiple times every night to pee!

These days, we ingest and absorb more and more toxins than ever before. Toxins are in our food, water and body care products. Don't let them take up residence in your precious prostate. Please read more about how to improve your diet in my other book, *The Prostate Health Diet*.

One of the main reasons I've written this book is to help you learn how to flush these toxins from the prostate.

Function 7: Erections

The prostate erection nerves are responsible for erections. These nerves trigger the penis to swell and harden with extra blood flow into it, producing an erection.

If these nerves, which attach to the sides of the prostate, get damaged then erectile difficulties are guaranteed. That is why many medical prostate procedures—surgery or radiation—have an unwanted side effect of erectile difficulties or impotence.

One relevant benefit of prostate massage is that it can stimulate these nerves thereby helping erectile function.

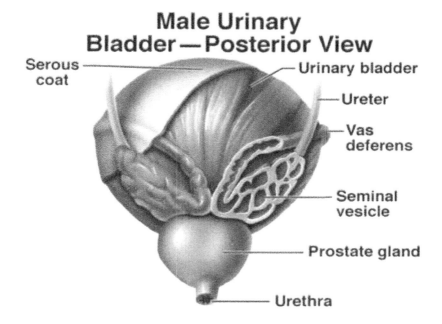

Male Urinary Bladder—Posterior View

Serous coat

Urinary bladder

Ureter

Vas deferens

Seminal vesicle

Prostate gland

Urethra

Function 8: Secretions

Prostatic secretions also play a valuable role by protecting the urethra from urinary tract infections, which as a result seem to be much rarer in men than in women.

Function 9: Valves

Just below the bladder, the prostate surrounds the upper part of the urethra tube, also known as the prostatic urethra. At this location, the prostate prevents urine from leaving the bladder, except when released by urination. It also prevents urine from damaging ejaculate during orgasm. It thus controls the flow of urine.

The prostate does this with two small muscles called sphincters. They act as gatekeepers with shut-off valves to control and regulate the dual-purpose urethra tube. These gatekeepers ensure the right fluids flow at the right time—urination or ejaculation. Not a bad design!

One sphincter is located where the bladder and the upper part of the prostate meet (the internal upper sphincter). When functioning properly, this sphincter prevents urination until it's time to go and stops seminal fluid from shooting backwards into the bladder during ejaculation. When damaged, semen is forced back into the bladder and eventually exits with normal urination. This is known as retrograde ejaculation and is another possible side effect of prostate surgery—no chance of getting a woman pregnant then.

The second, external lower sphincter is at the base of the prostate and is subject to our control. This sphincter prevents dribbling after peeing and is how we can voluntarily delay urination when inconvenient to go.

Incontinence occurs when control of either sphincter is damaged and urine leaks or flows uncontrollably, thus forcing many men with prostate problems to wear adult diapers.

It's easy enough to voluntarily control the lower sphincter and to stop urine or semen from exiting if you have enough Kegel muscle control, the ability to squeeze the flow shut. Either one of these sphincter muscles will block the urine until the urge to pee happens and the timing is right to release and let the urine flow.

Prostate exercises and massage can really benefit weaker sphincter control and thereby benefit your prostate health and sexual prowess, too.

An enlarged prostate or BPH can squeeze the prostatic urethra tube and the upper or lower sphincter, making urination difficult with a host of unpleasant, uncontrollable symptoms. BPH surgeries that remove part of the prostate can easily have side effects of incontinence or retrograde ejaculation.

Function 10: Hormones

The prostate gland contains a crucial enzyme, 5-alpha-reductase. This enzyme converts the hormone testosterone in the body to DHT (dihydrotestosterone), which is at least ten times more powerful than simple testosterone. This potent hormone DHT has several purposes including male sexual drive and function. Over time, a build-up of toxins in the prostate may negatively affect the production of this enzyme, which is then responsible for the declining sex drive in men as they age.

DHT and testosterone have mistakenly been targeted as guilty hormones in prostate problems rather than the excessive rise in modern male estrogen levels, which often leads to medical interventions with serious side effects including lack of libido.

Estrogen levels rise because of the prevalence of estrogens in factory foods, commercial meats and dairy, and estrogen-mimicking chemicals present in body care and household products. It's even found in municipal water and some plastic food packaging and store-printed receipts.

Conclusion

With such a complex gland having so many functions, prostate disease can wreak havoc on a man's health. Men would be wise to do all they can to enhance the health of their prostate—an unhealthy prostate can have an enormous impact on sexual function and simple daily urination.

The prostate is a powerhouse: a remarkable gland with huge repercussions on a man's quality of life!

Chapter 2
Benefits of Prostate Massage

Prostate massage moves stagnant fluids out of the prostate and provides a powerful health benefit for the gland. Prostate massage can also be an amazing sexual technique.

By sitting all day, as most men now do, we restrict the flow of blood to the prostate. This is one of the causes of our prostate troubles, especially when combined with all the other factors discussed in my book, *Healthy Prostate,* such as diet and exposures to chemical toxins.

Prostate massage is great for your health and pleasure. It can be done both externally and internally. It is something for men to use by themselves or for their partners to do with them. It can be done with or without sexual intent, and I cover both in this book. For now, let's talk about it just from the health point of view.

Prostate massage, both internal and external, is a wonderful technique to learn. Why? Because massage increases prostate health by improving blood circulation within the prostate and by removing stagnant fluids by releasing prostate fluids.

External prostate massage is a great way to reap the benefits of massage but is unlikely to remove as much stagnant prostate fluids as internal prostate massage. Nevertheless external prostate massage is well worth doing.

Prostate massage therapy is the name used for therapeutic prostate massage, which is done internally.

Prostate massage was a standard procedure until about 60 years ago. It was quite common for a doctor to provide internal prostate massage in the case of an enlarged prostate or of prostatitis. This technique would often provide the relief needed for either of these conditions.

With the advent of modern antibiotics, the practice was abandoned. Too bad, because in many cases the antibiotics do not work for the condition. Then the practice ebbed away, although the benefits are still acknowledged among doctors.

These days the practice of prostate massage is making a comeback as men learn the benefits for overall prostate health and sexual fulfillment.

You might enjoy this article: "Prostate Massage Reduces Cancer Risk" (goo.gl/zi8fwv).

You may be able to find a prostate massage therapist in your area. This may be a good option for you if you do not want to learn how to do it yourself, but it is easy to learn.

Removal of stagnant fluids from within the prostate can easily happen without an erection or ejaculation. With internal massage, sometimes fluid can come out of a non-erect penis.

If you are doing it alone or with someone you trust, you can choose to add sexual stimulation to the massage. Because the massage helps empty the prostate of fluids, the orgasm experienced with sexual prostate massage can be truly enjoyable and intense. I discuss sexual massage further in Chapter 4.

Prostate massage makes a big difference to your prostate health either in preventing prostate problems or in helping to heal a prostate condition. Massage benefits you and your prostate in two significant ways:

1. It increases freshly oxygenated blood flow to your prostate.
2. It releases fluids and flushes toxins.

With prostate massage, a wonderful sensation may flood the prostate area; you may or may not experience any release of prostatic fluids. Men with a prostate condition, such as an enlarged prostate, may release none or only a few drops of prostate milk.

You should ask your health practitioner for advice on whether prostate massage can be beneficial for you. There have been instances where vigorous massage has caused more harm than good. That's why careful and **gentle** prostate massage techniques are essential. (See Chapter 4 for more about safe prostate massage.)

External prostate massage is the easiest to do and can be as simple as doing Kegel exercises, which are discussed in depth at the end of this chapter.

Prostate Milk

Why is it called prostate milk? When you massage the prostate non-sexually, the only fluid that is released is that which is made right in the prostate.

When you have a full sexual orgasm, this fluid is added to the ejaculate that is formed in other reproductive organs (the testes and the seminal vesicles).

Prostate milk protects the sperm and enhances the chance of impregnation in women. This fluid is a naturally milky-colored fluid and thus is known as prostate milk.

Prostate milking massage, prostate drainage and prostate gland flushing are all terms used to describe prostate massage because it is often possible to excrete these prostatic fluids from the prostate without an erection or orgasm. This fluid does not contain any sperm from the testicles.

When men ejaculate during orgasm, the sticky semen contains

1. sperm from the testicles,
2. fluids from two small glands—the seminal vesicles—located right beside and above the prostate, and produce about 60% of the seminal fluid, and
3. alkaline fluids—prostate milk—from the prostate, about 30 to 35% of the semen.

Prostate Exercises

Prostate exercise strengthens the prostate and helps cleanse it of toxins by increasing blood flow through it. After all, the prostate is both a gland that secretes seminal fluids, is a muscle that pumps it out for our pleasure, and is a filter that removes toxins.

As the prostate is both a gland and a muscle, prostate exercises help keep the prostate toned. So exercising the prostate makes good sense.

An added bonus of prostate exercising is that it helps you control ejaculation and the duration and strength of your erections. Nice bonuses. Sign me up! ☺

Prostate exercise happens by engaging your pubococcygeus or PC muscle. Kegel exercises, or pelvic floor exercises, are the name used for both men and women to strengthen the PC muscle. It stretches from the pubic bone to the tailbone, supporting the inner organs of the pelvic area and the function of the sphincter muscles (anal and bladder sphincters).

In men, Kegel exercises also help to squeeze the prostate gland, which allows more blood to flow through it and helps to cleanse it.

That's why prostate or Kegel exercises for men are recommended for treating prostate conditions like enlargement, from benign prostatic hyperplasia (BPH), and prostatitis, inflammation of the prostate. Kegel exercises can also be used for treating urinary incontinence because these exercises strengthen the bladder sphincter.

For women reading this book, you can do the same exercises. Kegel exercises will strengthen your pelvic muscles and organs. As a result it will heighten your sensations during sex. Within 2 weeks, you will be able to squeeze your vagina muscles tight. I will leave it to you to imagine the pleasurable benefits of this skill for you and your partner!

Do you know how to squeeze your PC muscle? It's real simple. Just squeeze your stop-pee (and stop-pooh) muscle next time you are urinating to stop the flow completely. That's what you want to exercise— your PC muscle. Just tighten all the muscles around the scrotum and anus. It automatically engages the prostate and you are on your way.

You can now do this exercise several times a day anywhere—while sitting, driving, walking, talking, or now while you are reading this book! Squeeze, hold, release. That's it. The world's easiest exercise and perhaps also the most beneficial! And only you know you are doing it!

To get the most benefit from it, you need to do sets. You can vary:

- the speed of the squeezes from slow to fast,
- the duration of the holding time,
- the number of repetitions, and
- the number of times during the day you do sets.

Beginner Level

1. Breathe deeply while doing the exercises, remembering to clench only the PC muscle.
2. Squeeze and release quickly 10 times. Do three reps with a 10-second break between them.
3. Squeeze and hold for 10 seconds. Do three reps with a 10-second break between them.
4. You've just done one set. Repeat for a total of three sets for the day.
5. Repeat this process every day for 1 to 2 weeks.

Intermediate Level

1. Breathe deeply while doing the exercises, remembering to clench only the PC muscle.
2. Squeeze and release quickly 20 times. Do three reps with a 10-second break between them.
3. Squeeze and hold for 20 seconds. Do three reps with a 10-second break between them.
4. You've just done one set. Repeat for a total of three sets for the day.
5. Repeat this process every day for 1 to 2 weeks.

Advanced Level

1. Breathe deeply while doing the exercises, remembering to clench only the PC muscle.
2. Squeeze and release quickly 30 times. Do three reps with a 10-second break between them.

3. Squeeze and hold for 30 seconds. Do three reps with a 10-second break between them.

4. You've just done one set. Repeat for a total of three sets for the day.

5. You can do a mix-up: squeeze 30 then hold one for 30 seconds.

6. Repeat this process every day for 1 to 2 weeks.

Master Level

This is a whole body exercise that strongly squeezes your prostate and stomach muscles at the same time. The breathing is advanced yogic breathing.

1. Breathe deeply, ideally in and out through the nose while doing the exercises.

2. You are going to squeeze not only the prostate with PC contractions but the whole body at the same time and in particular the stomach muscles.

3. Bend your legs into a semi-crouch, legs hip width apart, hands leaning on your knees, arms straight, fingers splayed downwards.

4. While breathing deeply through the nose, arch your back into a concave shape: bum out and up, head up, and small of the back arched so the belly extends to the ground.

5. Then, come upwards into a quarter crouch, with knees still bent a bit.

6. While breathing out powerfully through your nose from the base of your diaphragm, arch your back into a convex rounded position, as hands move up to mid-thigh level, arms straight, head downwards.

7. Pretend you have a lemon inside your stomach, and you need to squeeze all the juice out of it by clenching and lifting your PC muscle upwards while pulling your stomach deeply inwards towards your spine.

8. Tighten (contract) every muscle in your body while pulling upon your kneecap muscles, thigh muscles engaged, and holding all the squeezes, energy moving upwards.

9. Hold for 10 seconds then release back down to the start position (see Step 3). Breathe in through the nose and repeat Steps 3 to 10 of the exercise.

NOTE: If your stomach muscles are not strong already, then 10 reps is way too many. It's not that you won't be able to do them but, 2 to 4 hours later, your stomach will be in agony. Start with three reps and work your way up to 10 over a couple of weeks.

Remember to do your prostate exercises every day. These are especially easy to do when you are waiting at traffic lights or watching TV. Put those down times to good use and your prostate will sing its praises!

Chapter 3
External Prostate Massage

As was mentioned earlier, external prostate massage is the simplest and easiest to do. Prostate massage can be simple prostate exercises done regularly (see the end of Chapter 2). In this section, however, we'll take it beyond the squeezing and add the massaging.

Benefits from external prostate massage could mean that your pain will subside, your sex life returns, and healthy urinating patterns are regained. You may wake less and less each night.

External prostate massage consists of direct pressure and gentle massage of the taint area (otherwise known as the perineum or male G-spot) either with the soft pads of your fingers or with a special device.

The perineum is generally a diamond-shaped area that includes both the anus and the genitals, and its boundaries vary. Keep in mind while giving a perineum massage that it's not just a superficial area; it's also quite deep. It includes the fascia and muscles in the center of the pelvic region.

Within this area is the male G-spot. Yes, you know about the women's G-spot and may have spent some time trying to figure out how to stimulate it, but how about your own?

The G-spot is located about one inch forward of the rectum towards the scrotum and is a key acupressure and acupuncture point. But let's not think about a needle there. Instead, imagine your own—or your partner's—fingers there instead. Or you can imagine a massage device doing the trick. A little later in the book, I delve further into one particular device that's used externally.

Always check with your doctor to see if prostate massage is for you. If so, be gentle and slowly build up the time that you spend doing this. Vigorous massage can be harmful.

Non-Sexual External Prostate Massage

Direct massage of the perineum—aka your G-spot—with oil while squeezing your prostate muscles is the simplest external massage. This 'double action' of external massage and squeeze is even more potent than just squeezing your muscles alone.

On a deeper level, the male G-spot is the prostate gland itself, accessed directly through the rectum in an internal prostate massage described later. For now, let's start with the external finger massage.

Finger Massage

All right, here are some tips.

1. Use some high quality natural castor oil (goo.gl/EITYCh) or almond oil (goo.gl/hG4V7s) to massage the perineum area while at the same time doing your prostate exercises, squeezing the pubococcygeus or PC muscle. The combination is very powerful and will bring much of the benefit of an internal prostate massage.

2. Find your male G-spot. Again, it's about one inch forward of the rectum towards the scrotum. If massaged during sex, the prostate is stimulated for double pleasure. Pressure on the G-spot can also be used to stop ejaculation if pressed deeply just before the tipping point.

3. Do the perineum massage gently at first and increase the pressure as you go along. Move in circles. Then deeply massage the G-Spot, all while doing your prostate exercises—squeezing and holding with deep nasal breathing in and out.

External Massage Device: The Prostate Cradle

You can use an external prostate massager like the **Prostate Cradle** (goo.gl/zXvquR). The Prostate Cradle is a wonderful invention that does the massage for you by just sitting. Highly acclaimed, this device is a natural and safe easy way to get the benefits of prostate massage.

It won't be as powerful as an insertion device but can be a good way to start. All you do is sit on it and move, and it does its massaging.

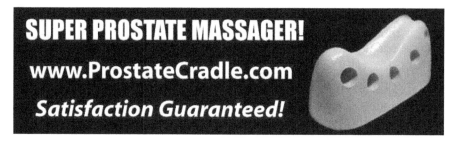

Read what the company has to say about it in a press release

After ten years of research and guidance from Medical Doctors the world's first anatomically correct, external prostate massager was created: the Prostate Cradle...

The Prostate Cradle was invented by a Certified Massage Therapist who was challenged with prostate health issues. His doctors recommended prostate massage therapy. However, at the time the only prostate massagers available were invasive. Traditional prostate massage involves rectum insertion. He knew there had to be another way!

The Cradle provides a revolutionary new way to massage the prostate: Simply sit on it! No movement or rocking is required. Body weight creates gentle pressure for a stimulating massage.

The Cradle is not like sitting on a bicycle seat. The unique anatomically correct shape avoids sensitive areas. The Cradle carefully reaches underneath the pelvic arch to massage the prostate and perineum area, also known as the "Male G-Spot."

It is important to note, dear reader, that the benefits of prostate massage accrue over time. If you have a prostate condition, it can take a week or two of massaging every other day before noticing the benefits. So be patient and give it a chance.

Chapter 4
Internal Prostate Massage

Internal prostate massage, or prostate milking massage, requires more effort but has maximum benefits. Why? Because the prostate gets stimulated and massaged much more directly through the thin anal canal of the rectum. Blood flow is enhanced and more toxin removal can happen.

Please note that internal prostate massage is done by inserting a finger or a prostate massage device gently into the rectum so as to get as close as possible to the prostate.

Internal prostate massage can be non-sexual or sexual as desired and chosen. I will cover both in this chapter.

Male prostate milking was the name given by doctors and urologists back when they did the prostate massage as a part of a healthy checkup for men. They used to massage the prostate in a non-sexual way to remove stagnant fluids and increase blood flow as a routine part of the digital rectal exam. (See the next section, "Internal Prostate Massage is not like the DRE.")

Enlarged prostates were often treated by doing prostate massage. The doctor's massage caused seminal fluids to flow—rather than squirt—out of the prostate, and from a flaccid penis, without sexual stimulation.

This is no longer standard practice and is considered alternative prostate massage therapy. However, conventional medicine still recognizes the benefits of therapeutic prostate massage.

Prostate massage is easy to learn, and massage devices make it safe and very effective. All you have to do is get over any hang-ups you have around the anus.

Anal stimulation is healthy. Just get clean, use lots of lube and read on about how to do it. The anus is the gateway to your prostate if you want to do internal prostate massage therapy.

Male prostate stimulation via an internal massage requires learning how to do it safely and with the correct techniques. The three basic ways of doing it are with

1. your finger or your lover's, or those of a practitioner who specializes in the technique;
2. a specially designed and very safe internal prostate massage device; and
3. an electronic pulsating prostate device, which is faster to use and easier.

Always check with your doctor to see if prostate massage is for you. If so, be gentle and slowly build up the time that you spend doing this. Vigorous massage can be harmful. (See the section below, "Safe Prostate Massage.")

Internal Prostate Massage Is <u>NOT</u> Like the Dreaded Digital Rectal Exam (DRE)!

Most men who have had a DRE, or Digital Rectal Exam, by a doctor or urologist have unfortunately experienced discomfort and often pain because of the very poor technique employed by most doctors.

If done properly and gently, the exam should be painless and quick. It is all a matter of proper technique, care and gentleness to give the anal muscles a chance to relax.

Let's face it—the first automatic response to the rectum being touched is to squeeze shut! If time is not given with very gentle pressure for it to relax, when the doctor inserts the finger it will hurt!

Too bad they are not properly trained. Always tell your doc to go slow so the muscle can relax before he pushes his finger in. In fact, a good doctor will ask you to cough, which can allow easier entry at the same time.

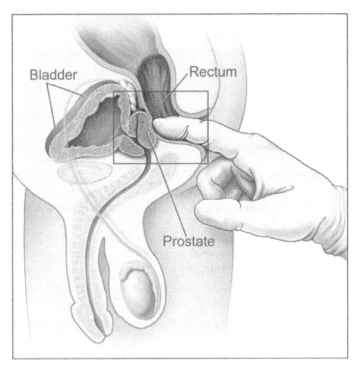

I am explaining this here so that if you've had a bad DRE experience, you can get over any negative thoughts you have about doing an internal prostate massage. Massage can be highly beneficial to your prostate health and extremely pleasurable, too.

It just has to be done properly.

When you follow my instructions below, you will not experience any pain or discomfort whether you use your finger, your lover's finger or an internal prostate massage device. In fact, it can be quite enjoyable.

Safe Prostate Massage

Here is how to massage the prostate safely, whether you are doing it yourself or a lover is doing it for you, with or without a prostate massage device. Please spend some time reading up on my tips below to avoid possible injury to your prostate gland, especially if you have a prostate condition.

When you massage your prostate, always be careful to be gentle. Gentleness is the key so as not to cause damage or to injure the tissues of the prostate. Never, ever use vigorous motion.

If you practice vigorous massage or use a lot of pressure because you think this will produce an even better massage or orgasm, you can damage the very sensitive tissues of your prostate. Remember your prostate is a sensitive gland and a pumping muscle.

The prostate needs only subtle massage pressure for optimum results. By doing your own massage at first, you can control this pressure easily. You need to learn how to massage with the correct techniques—first, to enter the rectum easily and, second, to massage safely.

Many men react negatively at first to the concept of internal prostate massage. However, once you know how to massage the prostate and you understand the benefits of proper techniques, you will change your mind.

Look, I know all about that! I thought the anus was for one purpose only—a visit to the can daily! And the thought of touching that part of my body—let alone inserting a finger or prostate massage device—turned me right off!

Also, my experience with the famous digital rectal exam was not pleasant. It always hurt. The doctors who did it were not adept at it and never allowed time for the anal muscles to relax. When done properly, with a few seconds for the anus to relax to the touch, then it is not at all painful.

If you do it yourself or with a lover, you have all the time in the world for the anal sphincter to relax to allow comfortable entry. That makes the world of difference. And lots of lubrication is essential.

Once I got over my anal hang-ups and fears, I realized how pleasant the feelings are and how beneficial internal prostate massage can be. Being clean down there is the first step in knowing how to massage the prostate. So shower first before beginning.

Non-Sexual Internal Prostate Massage

In this section, we'll cover massaging with a finger, using prostate devices and working with a partner. Although I describe how to do it yourself, your partner can follow the instructions to do it for you if you want. Learning how to milk the prostate is easy and will reward you with increased health.

You can use your first or middle finger or a special massage device that is designed for optimum prostate massage. These are discussed in detail below.

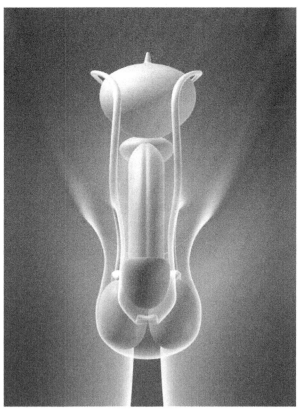

Under the big bulb above—your bladder—sits your prostate gland. It is filled with nerves and muscle. Attached to it are the prostate erection nerves that control your erections.

Finger Massage

Here is how to do internal prostate massage with your finger:

1. Make sure you have had a recent bowel movement so your rectum is completely empty.
2. Have a hot shower or bath to get clean or even a sitz bath to relax your pelvic muscles.
3. Make sure your fingernails are very smooth and short.
4. Wear a good quality latex glove (available at all pharmacies).
5. With a towel beneath you, prop yourself up with some pillows on your bed and with knees bent up, or lay on your side with knees bent toward your chest.
6. Apply a thick lubricant—KY jelly or personal lubrication (goo.gl/ZkeUay) or a natural castor oil—liberally to your fingers and anal area.
7. Gently press the pad of your middle finger against the anus so it starts to relax.
8. Move your finger gently in a tiny circular motion.
9. Take your time to relax. More time is good as it relaxes our usually very tight anal muscles. Enjoy the sensations. Take at least several minutes at this stage. There are many nerve endings here, and once you get over your mental up-tightness about this area and your muscles relax more and more, this alone will be very pleasurable.
10. After a while, slowly increase the pressure always allowing the anal muscles to relax as you then push a bit firmer until your finger starts to enter. You can also cough and at the same time push gently inwards. The coughing pulls inwards.
11. It is all about the correct angles to find the easiest way in. The pad of your finger should be facing forward—towards your front—as you find the way in. Move it forward and back to find the easy entry point. Once you get the right angle, it will slide right in an inch or two if you have enough lube.
12. At first, you may feel unused to the feeling, just because it's unusual. Take some slow deep breaths and let your body relax. It will adjust. Just relax and allow the feeling to unfold.
13. After a while, squeeze your sphincter muscles gently—this action will help move your finger in the last bit. Go slow while you get used to the sensation of having your prostate massaged in this way.
14. With your finger, press it gently upward (toward your navel) until you feel the prostate.

Now move the finger forwards and back in a "come hither" fashion as if you were beckoning someone, always slowly and gently. Gentle is the key so as not to cause damage or injure the tissues of the prostate. Never, ever use vigorous motion. Combine this with the squeezes for added benefit.

15. Being very gentle is essential, especially if you have a prostate condition because too much pressure can be too much for the prostate and can injure its very delicate internal structure of membranes. So always be gentle, never vigorous.

Do your Kegel squeeze exercises or "stop pee" muscle contractions to do the massaging motion as you gently move your finger at the same time.

16. Eventually, you may start to see some fluid (prostate milk) escaping your flaccid penis (a few drops or more). It does not matter if any fluid comes out, the massage is still very beneficial (see note below).

17. After 5–10–15 (less time at first) minutes, slowly remove your finger. Keep in mind that you can build up the amount of time that you massage your prostate for. At first, start with 5 minutes or less, then maybe 10 the next time, then 15. Slowly remove your finger when you've reached the maximum.

NOTE: This is an important piece of information—if you have a prostate condition, you can do the massage but find that no prostate milk comes out.

This is normal especially if you have an enlarged prostate. So do not be worried! You are still increasing the blood flow. You are still moving stagnant fluids and some fluid will move out later on as it works its way out and becomes part of your urine flow. Often, after the massage, you will excrete some fluid.

Another option is to use a prostate massage device. One of these can work well, too, and has some advantages as you will see next.

Prostate Massage Devices

I much prefer a prostate massager device. They are quite effective. They are specially designed to use your pubococcygeus or PC muscles in order to easily apply the right amount of gentle massaging pressure to the prostate.

A prostate massage device has at least two key advantages:

1. Safer: why?
   a. Because they can only go in so far, which is not too far that they can cause too much pressure and risk damage to the prostate gland;

b. Unlike a fingernail left untrimmed, it cannot cause any scratching of the gland; and

c. The right amount of massage pressure is used by doing the Kegel squeezes as described in the instructions and my tips below.

2. Better: why?

More territory is covered getting to spots that a finger will be unable to reach, thereby providing the benefit of more circulation and fluid release.

These are truly wonderful inventions that make internal prostate massage easy and very safe to do.

You can choose from two basic types of massage devices:

- Sonic prostate massager: a vibrating device (goo.gl/kvczqO)
- Pro-State prostate massager: a non-vibrating device (goo.gl/hB3lLs)

The Pro-State Prostate Massager: For a Healthy Prostate and Heightened Sexual Orgasms

We are lucky today because a new invention has made it possible for men to do a prostate massage by themselves that works much better than with the third finger or a lover's finger.

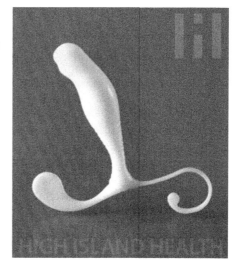

A key benefit of the device is its ability to reach more of the prostate gland than you can with your finger. It has a bigger area specially designed for maximum stimulation.

The Pro-State massager really takes prostate health and male sexual stimulation to a new level. In the picture below, you can see the perineum abutment is on the left, and the handle for insertion on the right side.

This picture shows what the Pro-State prostate massager looks like (goo.gl/hB3lLs). The tab on the left presses against your perineum (the key external male G-spot between your anus and scrotum), which stimulates your prostate. The right handle helps with insertion. The shape is designed to stay inside once inserted, and the tip massages both the main part and the side of the prostate.

The manufacturer says,

> The Pro-State prostate massagers are specifically
> designed for effectiveness and ease of insertion. Once
> inserted into the rectum, the anal sphincter naturally
> pushes the Pro-State up toward the prostate gland and
> the external arm of the Pro-State pushes up against
> the perineum.
>
> Prostate massage is most effective when pressure is
> applied simultaneously to both of these areas.
>
> Contraction and relaxation of the anal sphincter pivots
> the Pro-State massager up and down providing a
> hands-free massage of the entire prostate.
>
> In addition to massage of the prostate, the Pro-State
> prostate massagers are the only prostate massagers
> that provide acupressure therapy on the specific
> prostate perineum point.
>
> According to the precepts of Oriental medicine,
> massage of this acupressure point is beneficial for
> optimal prostate health and sexual function. The Pro-
> State prostate massagers combine these massages into
> one sophisticated method simultaneously, thus
> providing an effective massage.

The Pro-State prostate massager has several features that make it so
effective:

- The Tab: The small tab on the left is positioned to touch the G-
  spot between the anus and the scrotum. As you squeeze the
  Pro-State, the prostate abatement tab also massages this
  external prostate massage point automatically. Two massages in
  one! This increases blood flow and toxin removal. Great design!

- The Handle: On the right side is the handle for use in placing the
  device in and out.

- The Shaft: It is carefully designed to be the right size so as to
  gently massage the prostate and to be the right length as not to
  go in too far, which would be unhealthy. It also is made so that
  it does not slip out once inside your rectum. By doing simple
  Kegel squeezes or prostate exercises (squeezing and releasing
  the sphincter muscle), you can experience hands-free massage.
  As you squeeze, the device is pulled in further and massages
  your prostate. When you release, it moves outwards a bit.

- The Tip: This part is exceptionally well designed to massage the maximum amount of the prostate's surface—way more than is possible with your finger. It massages two sides of the prostate, actually, through the thin anal canal wall.

RELAXED SPHINCTER　　　　　**CONTRACTED SPHINCTER**

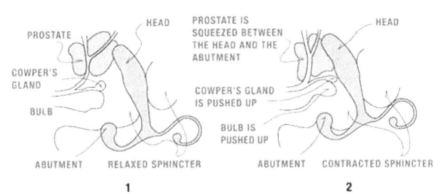

1　　　　　　　　　　　　　2

If you have never tried a Pro-State massager, it is well worth trying. The trick to using them is to apply lubrication liberally. It is really easy to insert when you follow my specific instructions below on how to massage the prostate with the Pro-State.

For prostate health, the Pro-State prostate massager excels at moving stagnant fluids and promoting blood flow in your prostate gland (goo.gl/hB3lLs). It does this safely and easily, simply because of its revolutionary and patented design.

Importantly, their design prevents injury as long as it is used correctly—meaning gently. You just cannot hurt yourself by using it correctly.

Do not be intimidated by the shape or size. They look a little weird until you understand how great a design it is.

The Pro-State prostate massager can be found at this URL: goo.gl/hB3lLs. While on the site, read the testimonials.

This massager will open up a whole world of pleasurable sensations and health benefits for you. Learn how to massage your prostate properly, and you will reap the rewards.

You may want to use the Pro-State massager for sexual pleasure; it brings you exceptional orgasms. Why? Because of the massaging action on the prostate. When combined with sexual stimulation, it will provide an amazing orgasm by releasing more ejaculate for a longer time period. Fun big time!

Not only is the device good for the prostate but also many men achieve success with erectile difficulties, probably because the prostate massage device moves stagnant fluids and stimulates the prostate erection nerves on the outside of the prostate.

Techniques for Using the Pro-State Prostate Massager

Here are my tips on how to use the Pro-State prostate massage device to get the most benefits while massaging internally:

1. Shower to get clean.
2. Lie on your back on your bed with good pillow support and a towel beneath you.
2. Always make sure you use lots of lubrication like KY Jelly or a natural castor oil. Yes—lots! It makes entry much easier and more comfortable. And it allows the prostate massager to move easily and smoothly.
3. With plenty of lube on the anus and device, simply apply some gentle pressure while moving it in a small circular motion to relax the anal muscles and sphincter. Take your time doing this. It makes it way easier once you have relaxed this area.
4. Make sure the small tab (perineum abutment tab) is facing upwards and the handle downwards
5. After a few minutes, you can press a bit firmer so that the prostate massage device starts to enter the anus. You can cough and, at the same time, push inwards.
6. The angle of entry is important. The line of least resistance is more towards your front than the back. Move it forward and back to find the easy entry point. When you get it right (facing forwards some) it will slip right in.
7. If you are having problems getting it in, then adjust the angle. When you get it right, it will slip right in a bit.
8. Once you have it in about a half-inch or so, adjust the angle until it finds the easy way in. When you have it right, a simple Kegel squeeze will slide it suddenly all the way in.
9. Now just relax and breathe and adjust to the feeling for a good 5-10 minutes.
10. Now you can begin with simple Kegel squeezes very gently— very gently.
11. You do not want to over-stimulate especially if you have a prostate condition.
12. Take your time, go slow and be gentle.
13. You may or may not expel some fluids from your flaccid penis. It does not matter. There will be prostate massage benefits and your prostate will be happy in either case. Often after the massage, you will excrete some fluid if none came before.
14. Please do not overdo it. Ten minutes to start, then increase to 20 to 30 minutes, which is plenty of time.
15. Gently remove the device.
16. Wash and clean thoroughly.

Prostate massagers are wonderful because they massage the prostate gland automatically while you simply lie there relaxed doing gentle Kegel squeezes.

You get the benefits of prostate squeezes and exercise which will thus improve overall sexual function. That's why this is such a good prostate massage device.

For those who are adventuresome, try using the device with sexual stimulation for amazing orgasms! For sexual stimulation, I leave that to your imagination or your partner's!

Remember that it is up to you how you want to do your massage. For men with a prostate health issue, the motivation will be prostate health. Prostate massage is a healthy way of benefiting your prostate.

For other men, sexual pleasure and enhanced orgasm will be their motivation, so go to Sexual Prostate Massage later in this chapter for more information.

Sonic Prostate Massager

The Sonic Prostate Massager is a portable battery-operated electronic device—really much more of an electronic medical device—that massages the prostate gently with pulsing sonic waves (goo.gl/kvczqO).

It can be much more efficient than a manual massager, much like a sonic toothbrush, with 40,000 massaging movements per minute, so it only takes 90 seconds of use once inserted, saving you a lot of time over the average 20 minutes recommended for the Pro-State prostate massager.

Exceptional in its design and ease of use, the waves help to move congested fluids out of the prostate gland and allow fresh blood and normal fluids to flow. You will observe the following effects in five short sessions, according to the manufacturer:

- Improves blood flow in your prostate gland.
- Improves lymph fluid flow, which helps to cleanse the blood in the affected areas.
- Stimulates nerve endings and improves erectile function.
- Strengthens and tones the prostate area muscles.
- Improves semen quality and flow.
- Strengthens bladder control, improves urination flow and relieves pain.

Relaxation of the prostate, as well as stimulation of the muscles, is a benefit of the sonic pulsations. Any inflammation you are experiencing could be reduced. In addition to metabolic processes being stimulated, you will experience an overall healing effect as nerve health may be restored and pain relieved.

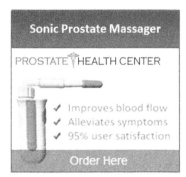

The Prostate Health Center makes the Sonic Prostate Massager (goo.gl/kvczqO). They are inexpensive and guaranteed; you can try them for 60 days risk free.

Many men have benefited from using these devices for their prostate condition.

This one is my choice for a simple non-sexual prostate massage for prostate health. I love the short time it takes and, as an added bonus, it is really easy to insert.

Because it uses electronic pulses from the battery, the massage head is smaller than the Pro-State, and this helps make it simple to insert.

Check out the feedback comments at the site and see what other men are saying about this great prostate massage device.

Techniques for Using Sonic Prostate Massager

You will need the following:

- some KY Jelly or personal lubrication (goo.gl/0N6U4b),
- some tissue,
- a towel, and
- a timer or watch.

Before I continue, keep in mind that vigorous prostate massage can be harmful. Think gentle, think slow. And check with your doctor first to see if it can help your particular condition.

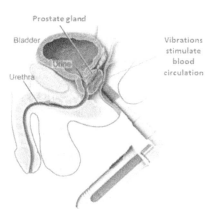

1. Have a bowel movement if you can.
2. Shower to get clean.
3. Place the towel on your bed and lie down on it with your back and head well supported by pillows, and knees up.

4. I prefer this position instead of the leaning-over-a-table method in their instructions. It is far easier and more relaxing.

5. Apply lots of KY Jelly or a thick personal lubricant to your anus and the tip of the sonic massager to make entry easy (goo.gl/0N6U4b).

6. Put some lubricant on your anus and on the massage head of the device.

7. With the handle in the up position, touch the tip to your anus and move it in a circular motion to relax the anal sphincter.

8. Slowly start pressing inwards, adjusting the angle of entry forward and backwards until it finds the easy way in. You can squeeze to help it do so.

9. Once it is in a bit, make sure your angle of entry of the tip is more upwards towards your front as this is the direction of the anal tube. Once you have the right angle, a little extra push will help it slide in for a total depth of around 2 inches.

10. Allow a bit of time to get comfortable with the feeling.

11. Once in, press the start button and time your massage for 60 seconds for the first time increasing to 90 to 120 seconds on future uses.

12. After 15 seconds, start moving the device by gently pushing up and down on the handle so the massage head presses against your prostate.

11. Move this back and forth (up/down/in/out/left/right) until the time is up.

12. That's all that is needed. Switch off and remove.

13. Do not surpass the time as too much stimulation defeats the purpose of the massage and will be too energetic for your prostate, and it could be harmful if you have a prostate condition.

14. Clean up the device head with warm soapy water.

15. Wait at least 48 hours before you do the next massage, maybe 2 to 3 times per week.

That's it! Now you know how to massage the prostate quickly and easily with this wonderful device. If you are doing internal prostate massage for sexual pleasure, keep all of the above tips in mind for maximum enjoyment.

Sexual Internal Prostate Massage

For those men who want to discover the added benefits of sexual prostate massage, a whole world of new sensations and skills awaits you.

Prostate massage has wonderful benefits for your prostate health. Prostate massage can also enhance sex if you want that! Somehow I think most men have an interest in that subject.

When sexual stimulation, such as masturbation or partner stimulation, is added to the internal prostate massage, the combination can lead to heightened arousal, an extremely pleasurable sexual response, and intensified and exceptional orgasms.

If you haven't yet discovered the world of sexual prostate massage, you may have been missing out on the best sex of your life.

That's quite a statement, but know that your prostate is your key to the best sex ever. Why? Because the prostate is designed to optimize your sexual function. That little prostate gland has a world of functions, but its secret is the best sex possible. And sexual prostate massage can add a whole other dimension to your sex life.

But wait for the sexual component until after you have done the prostate massage alone for 10–20 minutes first. This way you get both therapeutic and sexual benefits.

Sexual prostate massage stimulates both the prostate itself and the prostate erection nerves. The prostate erectile nerves that you'll be stimulating are responsible for the swelling and hardening of the penis. If you want to, pleasure yourself the way you would normally. In addition, do a sexual prostate massage for the key to your intense pleasure.

When prostate milking massage is done with sexual stimulation in mind, the amount of fluids in the ejaculate is usually increased and is one of the reasons prostate massage and sexual orgasm is so wonderful! Let's talk more about the orgasm.

Prostate Massage Orgasm

When you do prostate massage with sex in mind—adding sexual stimulation to the massage—the orgasm is much longer and more powerful than a regular ejaculation. Most men would like this added bonus! You have got to try it to believe the difference.

Rather than prostate massage be solely for therapeutic purposes—blood flow and stagnant prostate fluid movement—the little-known male G-spot can and will shower its blessings with truly wonderful orgasms that will knock your socks off (if you're still wearing them) when you finally release.

And there are advanced techniques—you can learn to have what is called multiple male orgasms! Not just for women!

I don't want to downplay the medical and healing benefits of self-prostate massage, but what we're going to focus on here in this section will be your guide to self-prostate massage orgasm, sometimes known as prostate milking (although traditionally milking described the simple extraction of prostate fluids from a flaccid penis for health benefits).

If you have prostate problems, check with your doctor first to see if prostate massage is ideal or potentially harmful for your condition.

You can do it by yourself or with your partner. Doing prostate massage yourself is probably the best way to start so you are in control and can go at your own speed. This way you can take the time to be gentle and relaxed so it is comfortable as you experience the new sensations.

You can relax fully and find out what works for you, and there is no danger of hurting yourself if you are gentle. And then you can reap the rewards.

When you do it with someone else, you'll discover that a great deal of surrender is necessary. It's an extremely intimate act and requires much trust and deep relaxation.

All of the muscles in the area eventually loosen their grip, including places you didn't even know you were holding stress and tension, such as the deep gluteal muscles. Often we only realize that these are tight and painful when a masseuse digs in to our butt cheeks.

Once you let go, however, you'll see that it all promotes such an incredible release—much more profound than most male orgasms. A prostate orgasm takes you to a whole other level.

If you have never explored the rectum for massage purposes, it is time to let go of possible negative feelings or thoughts about this part of your body.

Advanced Thai Technique

This video shows a Thai master discussing prostate massage (goo.gl/JBJ4h1). He is a master of the body's energy flow; it's a thorough and non-sexual prostate video. You will learn a lot watching it, including some excellent self-massage tips.

Video Techniques for Pleasurable Sexual Prostate Massage

If you want to watch an excellent DVD instructional and educational video, check out the DVD at this URL: goo.gl/kbcv7l. It uses effective techniques on lifelike replicas so there is no pornographic content, but it does contain explicit detailed tips and effective techniques for exceptional massage using lifelike replicas:

Discover the techniques and strategies for skilled, confident prostate massage. Learn relaxing warm-ups, arousing external strokes and internal prostate stimulation. You will be on your way to enjoying stronger erections, deeper pleasure, and more powerful orgasms... You will quickly learn how to stimulate your lover's complete sexual system—so you can turn off the video and turn on your lover!

Tantra and Taoist Prostate Sex Practices

In Tantric (India) and Taoist (China) advanced sexual practices, the prostate was an area of the man's body that had to be mastered to control ejaculation and to prolong orgasm or to develop inner orgasm.

The longer you can build your sexual energy, the more intense lovemaking is. In the end, you can choose to ejaculate or not.

Breath control is the key. When the breath quickens, you can slow your breathing through your nose to slow down arousal in order to prolong sex. By focusing on long slow breathing—in and out only through the nose—the sexual energy moves up the body and thus delays ejaculation.

And Tantric or Taoist women always knew that to insert a finger during lovemaking added a huge degree of pleasure with the added benefit of being healthy for the prostate. Of course, she would have to be trained to use just the right amount of pressure—a very gentle one—so as not to damage the prostate.

So follow the instructions for non-sexual prostate massage, whether with a finger or a device. After doing non-sexual health promoting massage first, add sexual stimulation to the equation and see what happens.

If you want the best for an exceptional male prostate orgasm with an erection, nothing beats the Pro-State prostate massage device described earlier (goo.gl/hB3lLs). It allows you to be hands free for your massage thus giving you the ability to play with your partner or yourself if you so choose!

Sexual prostate massage enhances erections by allowing extra blood flow into the base of the penis during arousal. The difference is that you now add sexual stimulation to the equation either by masturbating or by your partner stroking you.

- Either by yourself or with a partner, use whichever method you prefer: finger or prostate massage device.
- Apply lube to the penis and scrotum areas and combine stimulation with the prostate massage. If using a finger, wear a latex glove.
- It is best to start the prostate massage first for a while, as you want the therapeutic benefit of the massage, too.

- Once you are ready, **always being very gentle** with the prostate massage, add the sexual enhancement, which will result in an incredible prostate orgasm as your whole body feels the stimulation inside and out.

Sex and Your Prostate

I wrote about the importance of sex in my book *Healthy Prostate*, but it's worth repeating here. Your prostate is the gateway to sexual fulfillment, and sex is very good for your prostate. As it is also a muscle, exercising it by ejaculating makes it pump and stay healthy. So regular sex or masturbation is good for your prostate while abstinence can lead to a build-up of more and more toxins.

Remember what we said about how complex the male sexual and reproductive system is? It is not just about a penis and gonads! Simply put, the prostate is the key to maximum sexual pleasure. A healthy prostate makes it possible to have great sex into your senior years.

Although the prostate's main function is to produce fluid that becomes part of the semen, during orgasm muscle contractions squeeze the prostate, which pumps fluid into the urethra to transport the sperm out the penis. A very pleasurable event! That's the technical part.

Advanced sex practice and secrets utilize the energy potential of the prostate to achieve sexual heights that most men don't even know about, let alone master.

In Chapter 1, we talked about how important it is for your prostate health to exercise your prostate by doing Kegel or prostate exercises.

The next time you do them, feel your perineum muscles as you squeeze and release. Actually touch them all the way from the scrotum to the anus and see how strong they are (or can be!).

Now find the acupuncture spot about half way between them. If you press in with your finger at this spot and move it a bit until you find the exact spot (you'll know), then you have got it right! This is the external male G-Spot. The internal G-Spot is the prostate itself that you can reach with a prostate massager, your finger or your loved one's finger through the rectal wall.

The external male G-Spot is a crucial sex tool. You can use it to control ejaculations by pressing it firmly before the point of no return. This way you can fall back from just before the peak and extend sexual orgasm, which can be separate from ejaculation. In advanced practice, it is possible to *injaculate* rather than ejaculate. See URLs in the Advanced Sexual Skills section below.

Remember that the sperm and semen produced by the testes and the seminal vesicles must enter the prostate through the ejaculatory duct. So squeezing or pressing the G-Spot helps to contain the ejaculate at source until the point of no return or until you choose not to ejaculate.

By strengthening the prostate muscles and thereby being able to squeeze the perineum muscles tight to contain the energy in your prostate, and/or by pressing and activating this G-Spot, you can delay and extend sex for a long time. You are using your prostate for maximum sexual gratification this way.

In fact, a very advanced sexual Tantric technique teaches how to control ejaculation by squeezing the prostate at the right moment just before the feeling to ejaculate... to achieve multiple orgasms. The energy is moved upwards inside the body.

Of course, the other benefit of the exercise is to make your erections stronger. Muscle is muscle and exercising a muscle strengthens it. When you do PC squeezes (Kegel exercises), the prostate and the inner penis or "hidden" penis (actually about 1/3 the length of the erect penis) gets stronger as well.

You can feel that part of the penis when you have a strong erection... it extends inside the perineum right below the prostate. I guess that is why this pubococcygeal muscle is nicknamed the "love muscle"!

How often should a man ejaculate? Depends on your health, your age and stamina. If you find yourself weakened, then you are coming too often. The goal is to move the energy through sex and to become rejuvenated.

You can have more frequent sex, but do not ejaculate if you find yourself weakened. Find your optimum level by how you feel. In advanced sex practice, you *injaculate* instead.

The old question, "Is sex good for the prostate?" is easily answered: YES! The key is not to over-ejaculate because if you find sex weakening you, you must learn these advanced practices to injaculate or not ejaculate at all, and then you can have sex as much as you want. So learn some of these techniques and keep squeezing your prostate muscles!

Advanced Sexual Skills

Here are some superb sites where you can learn more advanced sexual skills and insights:

> ***Multi-orgasms for men:*** *"Any man can become 'multi-orgasmic.' It only requires a basic understanding of male sexuality and certain techniques. Most men's sexuality is focused on the goal of ejaculating, rather than on the actual process of lovemaking. Once a man becomes multi-orgasmic he will not only be able to better satisfy himself, but also more effectively satisfy his partner." Read more at "Multiple Orgasm" (goo.gl/SCfPvn).*

Sacred spot massage: *"The G-Spot or Sacred Spot of a man is his prostate gland. Tantric philosophy considers the G-Spot a man's emotional sex center. Massaging the man's prostate releases tremendous amounts of emotional and physical stress." Read more at "Sacred Spot Massage" (goo.gl/wxGvAj).*

Tantra 101: *"Always remember to breathe! Breathing is such an important part of Tantric sexuality. The deeper you breathe the more you'll be present in your body and out of your analytical mind, and the more you'll both feel! Now this may sound far-fetched. What does deep breathing have to do with pleasure? Well follow the logic here. Tantric masters know that the deeper you breathe the more relaxed you get. The more relaxed the body gets the easier the blood flows, the more blood goes throughout your body especially to the skin and underlying tissue, the more receptive the nerve endings are to pick up the stimulation." Read more at "Tantra 101—Not Just For Men" by C. T. Lamborne (goo.gl/AJxuGr).*

Tantric Ejaculation Mastery: *"Ultimate Ejaculation Mastery teaches you to separate ejaculation from orgasm by infusing your whole body with that glorious energy. When you learn the orgasm mastery formula, you can avoid the contractions that initiate the emission of semen. When you're super turned on, you can still have those pelvic muscle contractions that feel so wonderful. That's what causes a dry or energy orgasm, a long series of slow pleasurable spasms with a rush of energy without ejaculating. I call these inner or implosive orgasms because you pump the energy back inside, circulate it over and over again, and reach higher and higher peaks." Read more at "Tantric Ejaculation Mastery" by S. Pokras (goo.gl/GWemR9).*

Tao of Sex 1: *"The fourth benefit of the Deer Exercise is that it builds up sexual ability and enables the man to prolong sexual intercourse. During 'ordinary' intercourse the prostate swells with semen to maximum size before ejaculating. During ejaculation, the prostate shoots out its contents in a series of contractions. Then, sexual intercourse ends. With nothing left to ejaculate, induce contractions, or maintain an erection (energy is lost during ejaculation), the man cannot continue to make love. But, if he uses the Deer Exercise to pump semen out of the prostate in small doses, pumping it in the other direction into the other glands and blood vessels, he can prolong* intercourse." Read more at "The Deer Exercise for Men" (goo.gl/k3s06t).

Tao of Sex 2: "In Taoist sex traditions, the man has his orgasm without ejaculating. He injaculates, instead. By pressing an acupuncture point located halfway between the anus and scrotum, the ejaculation can be reversed into an improved orgasm and the semen is recycled from the full prostate and reabsorbed into the blood. This point is known as the Jen-Mo acupuncture point or the Lion... When the Jen-Mo point is pressed just prior to an anticipated ejaculation, the energy goes up into the body through the meridians which originate at this point, instead of going out of the body as it does during ordinary ejaculation. Done in this way, the man still feels the pleasurable sensations which come with the pumping of the prostate, and he still experiences an orgasm. He continues to press this point until the orgasm, or 'injaculation,' is complete... With depression of the Lion, it may take as long as five minutes to empty the prostate. This results in a five-minute long orgasm!" Read more at "Injaculation vs. Ejaculation: Prolongation of Arousal and Longevity" (goo.gl/o6Zf86).

Chapter 5
Prostate Massage Resources

Dear reader, this section summarizes some of the material already presented and adds some new info links to other resources useful for some men. You can learn a lot just by reading about some of the programs without even buying their product.

Prostate Innovation

Precision Medicine

If you have a prostate condition that has been a serious health challenge for you, and you want to avoid the many common medical procedures that have some risky side effects of incontinence or erectile difficulties, then this major innovation may be worth investigating.

This Chinese urology clinic (3DProstateCure.com) has developed the leading edge of non-invasive, non-surgical prostate procedures for prostate diseases and many erectile problems.

It is the only prostate clinic that I know of in the world that can accurately diagnose the exact causes of your problem and then has the knowledge and skill to alleviate it with targeted injected medicines.

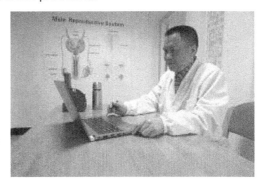

It is not a quick fix as it takes weeks of treatment time and healing after the treatment. But it works.

This remarkable prostate clinic changes everything we know about what causes prostate diseases and how to cure them.

From its site:

> The effectiveness of the 3D Treatment protocol is a result of three critical factors: (1) a full set of laboratory tests and examination procedures to determine the causative pathogens and pathogenic cells and locate the lesion tissue sites. (2) a local injection introduces the most effective treatment and unblocking medicines directly into the lesion tissue sites to kill the causative pathogens and pathogenic cells, and (3) a proprietary unblocking formula to clear blocked passageways and discharge toxic substances.

Dr. Song's 3D Prostate Clinic is perhaps the world's best natural clinic curing 95% of prostate cases, including many very complex ones.

Modified from acupuncture, this breakthrough uses no surgery, no toxic pills, just targeted precision medicine injections into the prostate of highly concentrated anti-bacterial, anti-viral and unblocking medicines that kills off the pathogens, viruses and bacteria that caused the prostate condition.

And with no side effects.

Just click on the image below to read all about his unique approach and methods to truly heal and cure your prostate problem, whether BPH enlarged prostate, prostatitis, or early stages of prostate cancer.

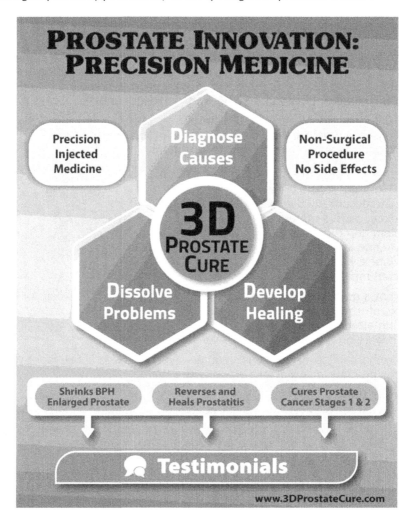

Devices

Sonic Prostate Massager— Vibrating

This is the best prostate massager to use if you want a therapeutic prostate massage and want it done fast (goo.gl/kvczqO).

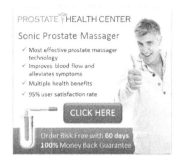

Pro-State Prostate Massage Device

The Pro-State is by far the best prostate massager to use if you have more time to relax and enjoy the benefits and pleasure of a prostate massage (goo.gl/hB3lLs).

By doing squeezes to do the massage, you also gain from strengthening your PC muscle. It is also ideal if you want to combine the prostate massage benefits with erotic sexual stimulation. The choice is yours in how you want to use it.

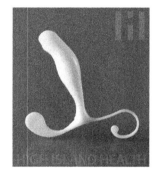

Lelo Prostate Massage Device— Vibrating

The Lelo is another excellent choice for both therapeutic prostate massage and great sexual stimulation. Find it at this URL: goo.gl/Yq5Oxh.

The Lelo has a smaller tip and thus is easier to insert. It has five differing stimulation modes plus controls for variable speeds and intensities. It's a bit more expensive but is quite the device!

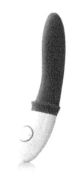

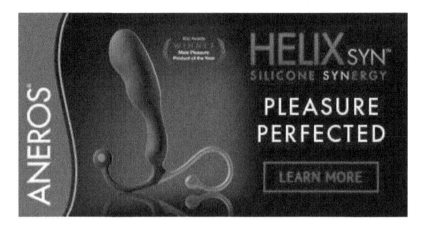

Info from its site:

Aneros products are hands-free, internationally patented devices specifically designed for prostate, or Male G-Spot stimulation (goo.gl/6RNYQD). Using no batteries or electronically induced vibrations, our products transform the body's own energy into amazing sensations. The mechanism is simple, but extremely effective.

With our products, a man can achieve strong, continuous full-body orgasms previously unattainable through conventional sexual techniques. These orgasms are so earth-shattering that they deserve a special nickname—The Super Orgasm, or as our enthusiasts prefer, The 'Super-O.'

A Super-O is entirely different from a traditional penile orgasm—it is characterized by pleasure starting from the lower abdomen that awashes the entire body in a state of bliss.

The man does not ejaculate during a Super-O. This means there is no 'recharging' or 'time out' period needed. Through practice, a man can have these orgasms, one after the other during sessions lasting for an hour or more at a time.

Even short sessions can feel long as our customers have reported that during Super-O sessions their 'beds shake uncontrollably' and they 'lose all track and sense of time.'

Aneros products can also be used during traditional sexual encounters (goo.gl/6RNYQD). During oral sex and traditional intercourse, when the man uses our products he will be harder, last longer, and have better control. His prostate will empty more fully during ejaculation, which means a more intense and satisfying orgasm.

This increased sexual performance is a great secondary benefit for the partner as well. Aneros is a great way to explore and expand your intimacy with your partner.

For these advanced sexual techniques and the Super Orgasm using the Aneros, go to Advanced Sexual Techniques (goo.gl/H0hbwc) and this URL (goo.gl/PvykDN).

Njoy Pure Wand

Njoy Pure Wand is both a male prostate massager and a female G-spot massager in one (goo.gl/D3mZUe). (Not quite sure if it can be used at the same time but maybe you can figure out how!). The small end is for men and the large end for women.

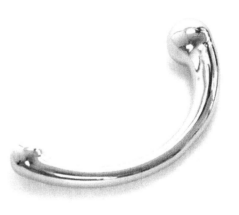

It is made from medical grade stainless steel. It is hand polished to a mirror shine and is completely body-safe. The ultimate sex toy?

Read the amazing 5-star reviews at Njoy Pure Wand at goo.gl/D3mZUe.

How to Nourish Your Prostate Gland

If you have started to make improvements to your prostate diet and your prostate health through prostate massage, you just may want to supplement with the most potent prostate supplement available today. I say that because one daily dose consists of about 6 to 8 times the quantity of ingredients than most other supplements available.

In fact, Prost-P10x uses the best quality sourced ingredients and makes no compromises (goo.gl/RvXaIx). The founder of the company successfully survived his own prostate health issues and made it his mission to educate men about prostate health. With Dr. Geo Espinso from NYU Department of Integrative Urology, the Prost-P10x's founder put the company together in order to research and make the best prostate supplement available for your health.

Each daily dose of 6 capsules comes in its own pack for easy use, which is a very convenient feature.

You will find cheaper products, but none will be finer or more potent nor will get the results of Prost-P10x (goo.gl/RvXaIx).

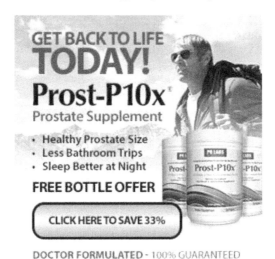

That's Craig, 53, the founder of the company in the picture below.

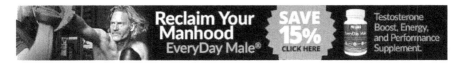

Other Books

More on Multiple Orgasms and Ejaculation Control

Alex Allman is a superb teacher of how to increase your sexual pleasure and your woman's as well. He has a remarkably frank and no-holds-barred way to inspire you and to teach his wonderful methods. You can find the free report at tiny.cc/dmadxx.

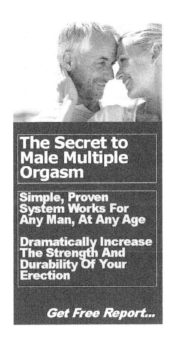

The Secret to Male Multiple Orgasm

Simple, Proven System Works For Any Man, At Any Age

Dramatically Increase The Strength And Durability Of Your Erection

Get Free Report...

Premature Ejaculation Problem?

Prostate exercises and massage should help you already. But if you want more tips and techniques, including physical and mental training that works, then check out some of these programs.

Premature Ejaculation Insights from Lloyd Lester:

> *Premature ejaculation is not some "gene" you're born with, the result of your penis size or a part of your personality that you can never change.*
>
> *Premature ejaculation is caused by specific things that you do before and during sex... most of the time without even realizing it.*
>
> *And if you want to last longer in bed you've got to take control of what you do before and during sex and start consciously doing things that will help you last longer.*
>
> *So below you'll find 6 tips to last longer in bed, which if you make into a habit of doing before/during sex, then premature ejaculation can become a thing of the past for you.*

1. Urinate Before Sex

   This is a simple trick most guys overlook. Before sex
   make sure you use the bathroom. If you don't then
   you'll have a full bladder which can put pressure on
   your genitals. And with pressure on your genitals
   you're more likely to experience premature ejaculation.

2. Master Your Pelvic Muscles
   There's a muscle in your genital area you can actually use to
   stop your ejaculation. This muscle is the same one you can use
   to stop the urine flow while urinating. Take the time to
   strengthen this muscle by "squeezing it" throughout the day.
   Eventually when it comes to sex this muscle will be so strong
   that if you squeeze it just before orgasm you can actually stop
   ejaculation from happening.

3. Use Slow Breathing
   Most men when it comes to sex out of excitement they end up
   taking lots of quick short shallow breaths. The problem with
   shallow fast breathing and overexcitement is that it can actually
   encourage premature ejaculation. Instead make a conscious
   effort to take some long slow breaths before and during sex,
   especially in and out through your nose. This is a great way to
   calm yourself down so you last longer.

4. Rub Her Clitoris
   A great tip to last longer in bed is to thrust really deep inside her
   (without hurting her obviously). And once you're in deep stay
   deep and just rub her clitoris with your pelvic bone. What's great
   about this sex technique is that it reduces your stimulation
   meaning you can last longer, but it gives her a ton of pleasure at
   the same time.

5. Masturbate For Longer
   When you masturbate you actually end up conditioning yourself
   for how long you expect your body and penis to last during sex.
   This means if you masturbate for a matter of minutes or even
   seconds then when it comes to sex you're not going to last any
   longer. In future, masturbate for much longer, as long as you'd
   like to last during sex. If you find yourself close to orgasm just
   stop for a minute, then restart.

6. Relax Your Muscles
   A dead simple way of lasting longer in bed is to just relax your
   muscles more. Normally you'll find that your muscles get more
   and more tense as you approach orgasm. When you notice this
   happening just allow your muscles to relax again. By consciously
   relaxing your muscles you can delay orgasm by several minutes.

To learn how you can end premature ejaculation for good, visit this link (goo.gl/m1FOvJ) or watch this video (goo.gl/6JoDL0):

Lloyd Lester has another program for getting erections if you suffer from performance anxiety.

Erection By Command

Getting it UP and staying UP: This is practically every guy's eternal quest. If the statistics are anything to go by, erectile dysfunction (ED) is the number ONE sexual condition that affects millions of men around the world. And a man's inability to get hard and stay hard during sex can quickly become a personal or relationship crisis.

While the avalanche of ED cures (pills, creams and even strange-looking devices) being peddled in late night TV shows and the back of sleazy magazine promise a quick, instant cure — most of them are costly, unreliable or even downright dangerous.

The truth is, most guys I know want a natural, reliable and permanent way to rise to the challenge. And this is what the program "Erection By Command" is all about.

"Erection By Command" is a professional guide designed to help men who suffer from erection difficulties—by re-conditioning the mind and body for instant arousal and erection.

"Erection By Command" sets itself apart in the male sexuality field by offering a unique, safe, and proven "mind- and body-based approach" to fixing ED. It appeals to guys who have to deal with psychologically-induced ED (such as those caused by sexual performance anxiety) and integrates sexual techniques with brainwave entrainment technology.

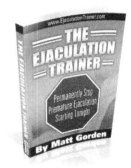

The Ejaculation Trainer (goo.gl/I5TVop) is another very impressive training guide to better sex. To give you an idea of the approach to premature ejaculation found in this book, the author, Matt Gorden, suggests these quick techniques to instantly last longer in bed:

While to gain long term and permanent control over premature ejaculation, men need to learn how to control their sexual response, retrain their ejaculatory reflex to naturally last longer, and learn some other critical information about ejaculation control.

However, there are moments where a quick, in the moment fix is needed when getting too close to ejaculation. Here are a few techniques that can be used to instantly last longer and delay ejaculation.

- *Focus on short, shallow penetrations. This will stimulate the vaginal entrance, where the majority of a woman's nerve endings are, giving them more pleasure. This will help women become aroused more quickly, which helps the man get the job done easier. Most importantly this will make it less stimulating for the man, effectively delaying ejaculation.*

- *Slow down the pace and take some slow, deep thrusts. This will decrease how much stimulation your penis is getting while not having to stop intercourse. When you are deep, try grinding your hips and wiggling your pelvic bone. This will reduce your stimulation even more while still stimulating her.*

- *Focus on your partner first before worrying about yourself. By making sure that she has an orgasm first, a lot of the pressure will be released, allowing you to relax some and not be so overwhelmed, which can affect how quickly you climax.*

- *If you do happen to ejaculate early, don't get discouraged and stop everything. Keep focusing on her and after a few minutes you will be ready for a second round. Most men last longer the second time around anyway and your partner will appreciate the extra attention.*

- *Switch it up and have her on top. Your penis will be less stimulated from this position, allowing you to regain control again. Ask her to go nice and slow at first to extend it even longer.*

- *There's no shame in having to just completely stop and compose yourself. If you can, try to keep playing with her while you calm down so she is not left lying there. Also, if she is still getting pleasured, she is less likely to notice that you pulled out for a minute or two.*

- *Put on a condom, not only do they immediately reduce stimulation to your penis, but they are a good safety measure.*

  While none of these are long-term solutions to relieving premature ejaculation, they are great quick fixes that can help men as they learn to control their arousal. When it comes to quick-fix techniques, these are nothing compared to the 18 quick-fix techniques and other information discussed in The Ejaculation Trainer (goo.gl/I5TVop).

Revive Her Drive

Susan speaks from experience and is superb at helping you understand your woman and how to get her going (an aroused woman is sure to help you with your arousal)...

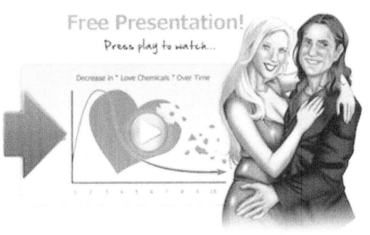

About the Author

Ronald M. Bazar, a Harvard MBA, is a natural health enthusiast and author of six books on the prostate including the comprehensive book on the prostate called *Healthy Prostate: The Extensive Guide to Prevent and Heal Prostate Problems Including Prostate Cancer, BPH Enlarged Prostate and Prostatitis* (goo.gl/pVZ6tr), which is available on Amazon, iTunes, Kindle and more outlets.

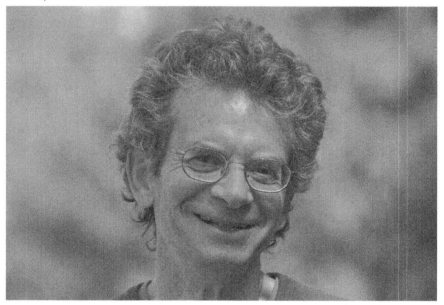

Ron: A "bit sweaty" after playing a long Ultimate Frisbee game at age 65!

Other Books by Ronald M. Bazar

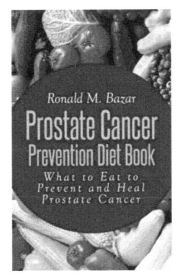

Prostate Cancer Prevention Diet: What to Eat to Prevent and Heal Prostate Cancer

(goo.gl/gF4vjX)

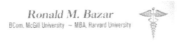
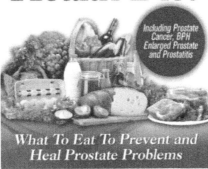

The Prostate Health Diet: What to Eat to Prevent and Heal Prostate Problems

(goo.gl/0UR6Zt)

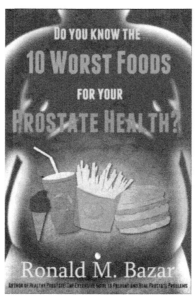

Do You Know the 10 Worst Foods for Your Prostate Health?
(goo.gl/AQm90i)

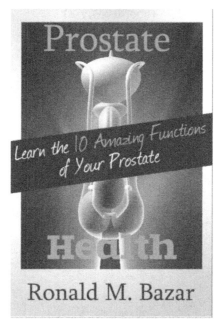

Prostate Health: Learn the 10 Functions of Your Prostate
(goo.gl/oyd4yu)

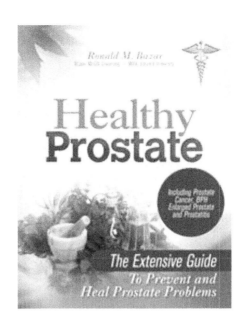

Healthy Prostate: The Extensive Guide to Prevent and Heal Prostate Problems Including Prostate Cancer, BPH Enlarged Prostate and Prostatitis

(goo.gl/pVZ6tr)

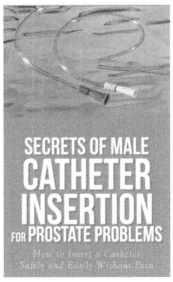

Secrets of Male Catheter Insertion for Prostate Problems: How to Insert a Catheter Safely and Easily Without Pain

(goo.gl/YbjyXA)

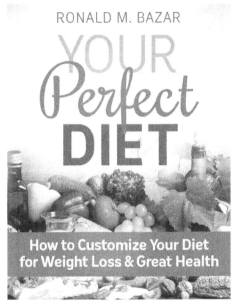

Your Perfect Diet: How to Customize Your Diet for Weight Loss and Great Health

(goo.gl/b30Xkk)

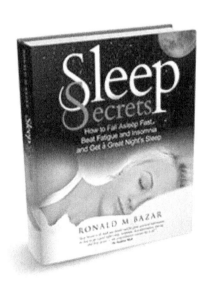

Sleep Secrets
How To Fall Asleep Fast, Beat Fatigue and Insomnia
and Get a Great Night's Sleep

(sleepsecrets.co/)

Made in the USA
Coppell, TX
19 February 2021